# The Fit Genie

Written by Author

## Ian McCranor

*A story for children . . . . A message for adults*

**Published by:**

# SanCo Media

**www.SanCoMedia.com**

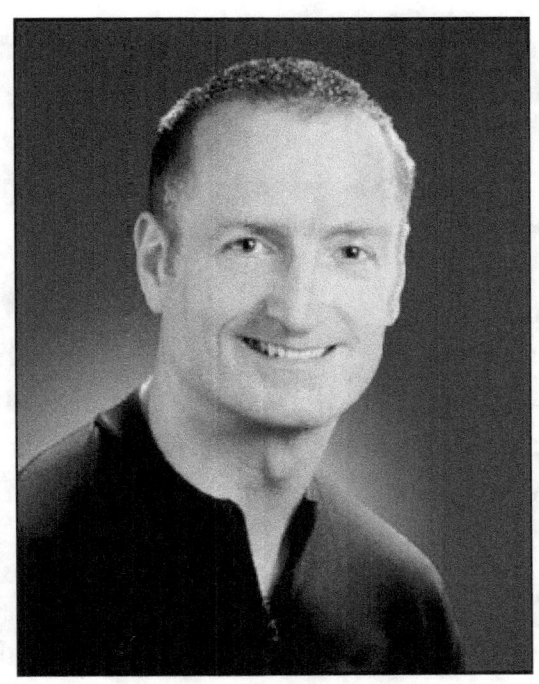

**Author Ian McCranor**

Ian McCranor is an ACE (American Council on Exercise) certified personal trainer and creator of TaeRobics.

As a former International karate champion and martial arts practitioner, Ian's unique approach to weight loss has many in the industry standing up and taking notice. Not one to shy away from controversy, Ian says, "You made your kids FAT, it's your fault".

Born and raised in Coventry, England, Ian's "its just human nature" brand of delivery is not only hard-hitting, but brutally honest and frequently hilarious.

Using a mystical being from another world (The Fit Genie), with the innocence of a child and the ignorance of a half wit, Ian can pose those awkward questions that often go unspoken: "So, if you don't like being fat, why are you fat then?"

As a former British nightclub bouncer over a fifteen-year period Ian witnessed what poor choice can do to a person. Drugs, alcohol and violence were just a small sample of vices that the human race seemed destined to endure.

"Why, when you were born with a fit healthy body, would you choose to create a fat, out of shape, unhealthy body? It makes no sense!" the Fit Genie says.

"The Facts/ The Truth can be a bitter pill to swallow, but our children are a gift from God and we should be doing everything we can to protect them, even from themselves," says Ian. Ian's first book in his Fit Genie series (The Fit Genie, "Freddy Dream") introduces parents to the genie and our children to their future…

# A MESSAGE TO ADULTS

*Please, read prior to reading to children!*

If you are fat, this story will make you angry; you will be upset by some of the content. I ask you to please take that anger and sit with it for a while as you debate the accuracy of what you are reading. My aim is not to offend, but I do a very good job of doing just that.

Fat people are a massive cash cow for the multi-million dollar weight loss industry. Any time you hear the words "easy" or "fast" combined with the words weight loss, you'll know it's a lie. Losing weight is very difficult; in fact, it is so difficult that the vast majority of fat adults will **<u>never lose weight</u>**. Once you are fat, you are fat for life. If the truth offends you, then you may want to leave this book where you found it. There are plenty of fiction books you may want to read instead. If, however, you want a straight-talking, no-nonsense approach to the subject, you have come to the right place. As I said, if you are fat, I guarantee you will be offended, but not nearly as much as when you learn what your friends and colleagues are saying about your fat backside behind your back. Read this story to your kids, and just maybe they won't trade in their health and happiness for a big, ugly gut, diabetes, heart disease and an early grave.

*This is a children's story with a serious message.*
*Omit or substitute dialog at your discretion.*

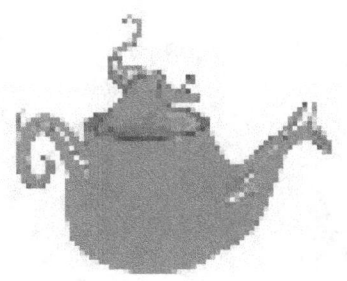

# *The Fit Genie*

This is about the Fit Genie.  The Fit Genie is from Great Britain, well, England, to be precise, so you may have a little difficulty understanding some of the things he says. Not to worry though; there is a lingo dictionary in the back of the book, so feel free to take a quick butcher's in the back from time to time. Oh, sorry, I've been hanging around the Fit Genie too long. 'Butcher's' means 'look.'

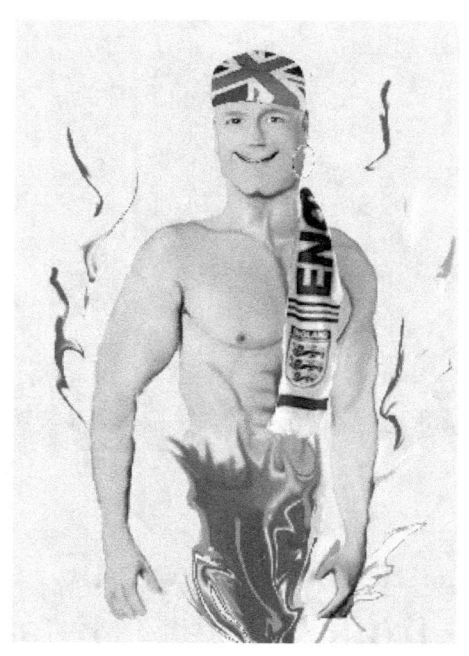

One other thing you may want to be aware of: this British Genie doesn't seem to possess the "insult filter." You know, you *think* something, but don't actually *say* it. Well, the Fit Genie is not like that. He can't stop himself, and he says the first thing that pops into his head. Really, he just says what everyone else is thinking.

This is the story about the time the Fit Genie made a really bad mistake when granting a wish. Genie tells the story much better than I do and with a way cooler accent, so I will let him continue.

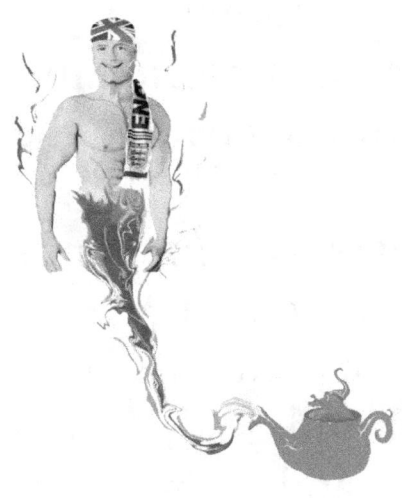

You humans are very hard to understand. I have learned so much about your species, but there is still so much I don't quite get and I don't think I ever will.

You are born with perfect health and with the potential to shape your bodies into a beautiful work of art. You have a clean, untouched canvas in front of you and a free will to create whatever you want. Why, then, when someone is given a choice to be slim, fit and healthy, would you choose to be fat, unfit and unhealthy? This was something that baffled my mind; at least it did until I uncovered the facts.

Many years ago, my lamp was found by a group of school kids. One of them picked it up, waking me from my kip. I appeared and said, "I am the genie of the lamp and I am here to grant you three wishes. Please use your first wish wisely, as once it has been granted it cannot be taken back or changed for something else. Once you have it, you're lumbered with it."

A snotty-nosed kid said. "Oh, wicked! What shall we wish for?" They talked for a while and decided that new bikes would be awesome.

"Genie, we would all like new bikes, please."

"New bikes? OK, what sort of bikes would you like? Racers, mountain bikes, BMX's, or maybe a chopper?"

A zit-faced kid said, "Wow, so many choices! How about if we all get one of each kind?"

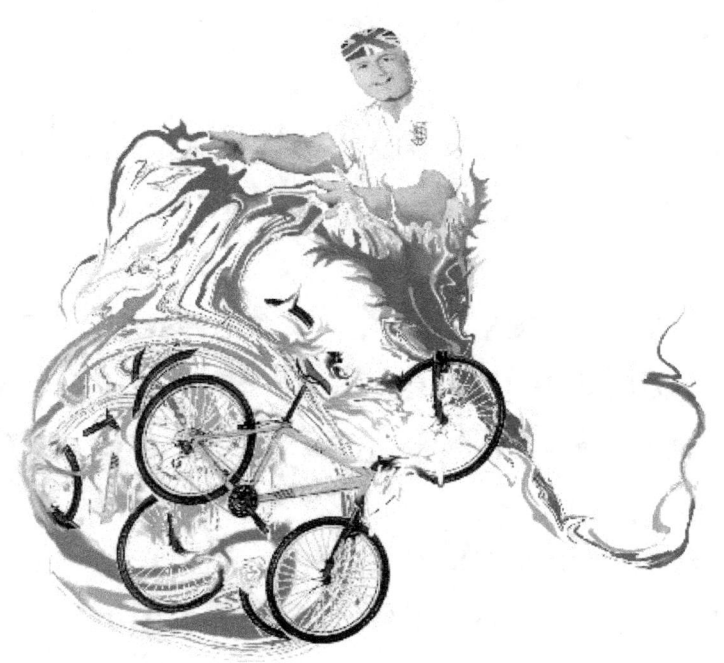

"Good plan," I said, and with a blink of an eye, they had their bikes. They got on their bikes and rode around for hours, stopping only when I reminded them they still had two wishes left.

"What would you like for your second wish? Please use your second wish wisely, as once it has been granted it can not be taken back or changed for something else. Once you have it, you're lumbered with it."

The kids had a bit of a chin wag. Then this boy (who I actually thought was a girl at the time because of his long, curly hair) said, "Video games… all the best video games please, Genie."

"Video games? That's a bit of a dumb thing to wish for," I said. "Why not wish for something like…hmm… new smart clothes, or some nice shoes… you know, something useful?" I think that comment annoyed a few of them because they started throwing stuff at me. Then a geeky kid called me an idiot, so I pushed him into a puddle. Anyway, they insisted on video games and I had no choice but to grant this wish; so, with a blink of an eye, their video games appeared.

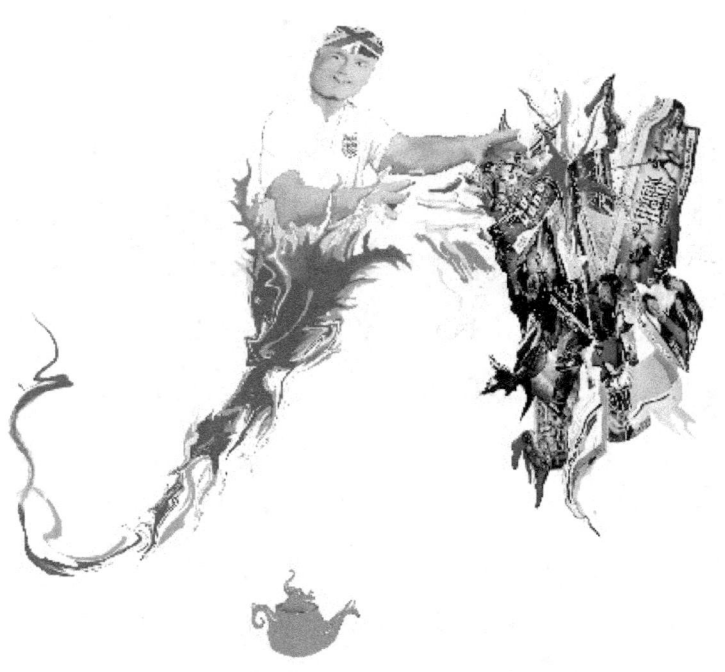

The kids left their bikes where they fell and went indoors to play video games for hours, stopping only when I reminded them that they still had one wish left.

"What would you like for your third and final wish? Please remember to use your last wish wisely, as once it has been granted it cannot be taken back or changed for something else. Once you have it, you're lumbered with it."

This is where all the trouble started. There was this fat, blobby-looking kid whose trousers were all baggy and almost falling down. (When he bent over, you could see his bum crack!) He was eating a huge ice cream cone, most of which he had all over his face. "OK, third wish, anyone?
Has anyone got any ideas?" Just as I got my last word out I saw a huge grin appear on Blobby's face, and I knew exactly what he was thinking!

"FOOD! How about loads of food?" I couldn't make out the exact words he used because he had just stuffed a large burger in his mouth, but I knew what he was asking for. The other kids all piped up.

"Yeah, we want pizza, cookies, pie and cake and make it so they keep appearing and never run out!"

"What kind of stupid, bozo, plonker wish is that?" I asked. "The bikes were a great wish. They get you outside in the fresh air and make you exercise. The video games are not what I would call a great choice; they can make you lazy, sitting around on your deaf and dumb for hours and hours; But all that food? Nope; not a good choice at all. You all know what will happen if you eat stuff like that, right? You will start to look like that heff!" (I was, of course, referring to the bum-crack kid.)

"Hey, who are you calling a heff?" he spluttered through his now cake-stuffed mouth. "I have a name, you know!"

"What is your name?" I asked, trying to divert attention away from this last wish. "My name is Freddy and I am not actually fat," he said.

Now I was confused. "You are not actually fat? So, what is all that hanging over your jeans, then? It looks like fat to me."

Freddy went on to explain, "I take after my family; they are all… well built," he said.

Again, I did not understand. "So, your entire family is fat then?" I said.

Freddy glared at me and yelled, "No, we are not fat! We are just a large-framed family!"

Oh, bless him, I thought to myself. He really has no idea! So, I used my genie magic and sent a truth-finding beam into his body. The beam came back and reported that, yes, I was right.

Looking very pleased with myself, I said, "Here, Freddy, this shows that you are indeed a big, fat, blobby git, and not big-framed at all! No need to thank me… just doing what genies do." Freddy stormed away crying. I thought they were tears of happiness, because now he knew what the big lump in his belly was. He could now do something about it.

One of the kids told me that I was very rude and I had upset Freddy. Another told me that I couldn't go around calling people fat. Now I was really starting to get confused.

"Okay, let me get this straight," I said. "Freddy's name is Freddy, right? So, is it okay to call him Freddy?"

The kids looked at each other, paused for a few seconds, and then one said, "Well, yes, of course it is, silly."

So, my next question was, "Freddy is fat, but I can't call him fat?"

They all yelled back immediately, "No, you can't!"

"Hmmm, I'm not sure I understand how this lying-to-yourself stuff works," I said. "But, back to your last wish, I have a great idea. How about a wish for fitness? Freddy, here is your chance! I can make you thin, fit, muscular and healthy. All of you, from this day forward, could be in great physical shape for the rest of your lives! Now *that* would be a smart wish!"

"Wow, that would be awesome!" said the geeky kid. "To eat what you want and never have to work out, but still be in great shape? Yes! Let's wish for that!"

"Oh, no, no, no, wait just a second there, Geek Boy! I can make you fit right now, but you will not stay that way unless you eat right and work out regularly. Yeah, that's right, all those fit people you see are that way because of healthy eating and regular exercise. It's not just luck, you know. So what do you say, do you want to be fit?"

Well, it didn't take long before Freddy answered, "What's the point if we can never eat our favorite foods? I like eating things like chocolate and drinking soda."

"I know you do, Freddy, that's why you are the size of a house," I said.

"GENIE!" the kids yelled.

"What? I never mentioned the word 'fat' at all! Ok, ok, I guess the word 'house' can't be used either! I am going to have to make a list!"
Curly Locks sat down next to me. "This is how it works," he said. "You can't mention anything at all that points out that people are fat. That's rude! It's very simple, Genie, anything to do with someone's size is out of bounds."

"OK," I said. "I am getting it. So, if someone were big and muscular, they would be offended if I said how great they looked?"

"Genie, you really are silly! No, that would be called a compliment, and yes, you can say that."

I was confused again. "So, the size thing actually depends on what the size is made of? If they are big from working out hard it's a compliment, but if they are big because they are lazy and fat, it's an insult?"

**"Exactly!"**

This begs the question: why, then, would someone choose to be big and fat? It just didn't make any sense to me whatsoever.

Trying desperately to understand this whole concept, I asked if the kids were actually aware that Freddy was fat, or did they not see what I saw?

"Oh, yes, we know how fat he is. We joke about him all the time; the way he waddles around panting for breath. The girls even call him Freddy French fry. When we go to the burger place we ask for a burger and Freddy fries. Even the people there know what we mean."

I was learning a lot about humans, and was now feeling bad about upsetting Freddy, so I thought it would be a good idea to go chat with him and see if we could start over. I wandered over to where he was sitting and told him I was sorry if I offended him; I was still learning how to talk to humans and didn't mean to be rude. He accepted my apology.

Then, I gathered the kids together and reminded them that they still had one wish left. I thought it would be a nice touch to let Freddy decide what the last wish should be, so I turned to Freddy and said, "So, Freddy French fry, what would you like for your last wish?" There was a stunned silence.

Freddy said, "What did you just call me?"

"Oops, give me just a jiffy," I said, and scooted out of there as fast as I could. I was met around the corner by Geek Boy. "Let me guess…he didn't know you call him that?" I said.

"No, he didn't. Now we are all in trouble," he said.

"I am never going to get to grips with the way you humans behave. You said you were all aware that he was fat and you called him Freddy French fry because of it. You lied to me!"

"No, Genie, we didn't lie.  We do all call him that, but not to his face! Everyone makes jokes about fat people, and everyone has names for people who are fat, but they don't say it right in front of them."

"Agghhh!    There are too many ridiculous rules to remember.  So, it's really ok to call people names and say things behind their backs, but it's only rude if they hear you.  Is that what you are saying?"

"Yes!...no!...oh, I don't know."

This conversation continued for quite a while, but human behavior just didn't make any sense to me at all.  So, I looked in my book of Genieology for information on humans. Here I discovered that humans lack the ability to be totally honest with each other, and lie to save feelings! The truth was often too painful to admit even to themselves.

Alas, I should have found this out before I put my big foot in it; if all I have to do is lie to humans, this should be easy. I now needed a lie I could tell to show the humans that I understood how it all worked. Suddenly, I thought of one!

"Freddy, my friend," I said, "I was mistaken. You are not fat at all; your big, flabby belly, saggy bum and bloated face is very attractive and nothing to do with being fat. It's just the way you were made, and there is nothing you can do about it. Your friends don't call you Freddy French fry, and when they go to the burger place they don't order a burger and Freddy fries. I would also have to say that without doubt you are the best looking, healthiest, non-fat kid I have ever seen. Go ahead, wish for all the food you can eat.  Stuff it down until you feel like you are going to explode, because the bigger you get, the better you look and the fitter you will feel!" (This was a wicked lie!  I was so pleased with myself.  I felt just like a human.)

Stunned silence, wide eyes and jaw-dropping expressions were the results.  I had obviously hit this one out of the park!  They were speechless; I am such a clever genie.

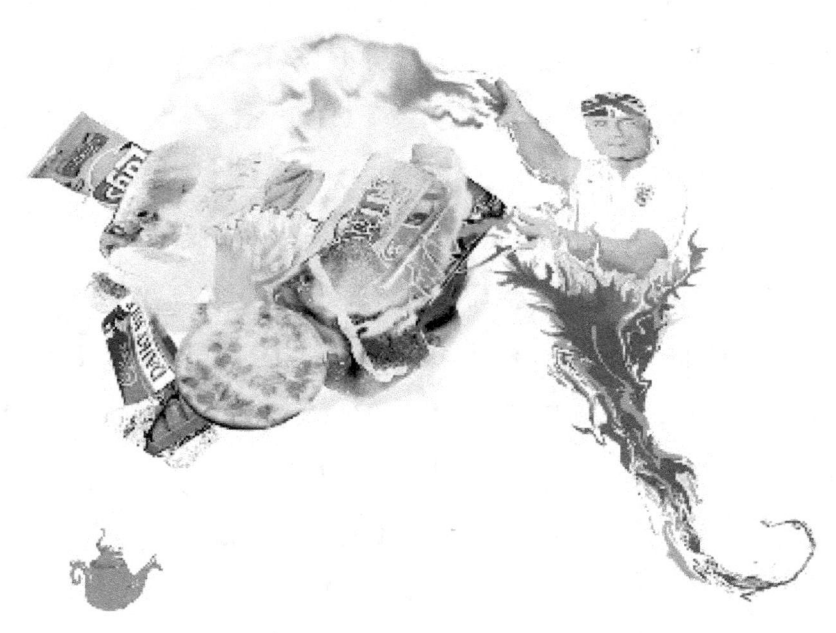

"So, back to your third and final wish, kids, an endless supply of your favorite foods, right? Yep, all this stuff is so good for you. You will not put on any weight; you will look good and feel great. Here we go!" And with a blink of an eye, their favorite foods appeared and re-appeared, magically replacing themselves fast and conveniently every time the kids took a bite.

I had now completed my duty and granted their three wishes. I stayed around for a little while, but watching kids stuffing in pizza, cake and soda while lying around playing video games made me feel a bit Tom and Dick, so I jumped back into my lamp and left them to it.

As expected, the kids ate and ate and ate. They became so fat that riding their bikes became a problem! So, they stayed in the house and played video games instead, and they ate… and ate… and ate… and became even fatter. Those fat kids became fat adults, who then became fat parents, whose kids played video games while they ate and ate and ate.

Many, many years had now passed when Lamp awoke me. "Genie, we have a problem," he said. He pulled out some pictures he had taken while on vacation. "Look, Genie, everyone is fat!" He showed me a picture taken on the beach. The entire beach was covered in flabby, soft, out-of-shape, ugly, disgusting rolls of blubber. Next was a picture taken on a cruise. I could not believe my eyes! These people gave a whole new meaning to the word 'fat'. This was no longer just about being unhealthy. This had now moved into the area of uncontrolled self-abuse. These people far surpassed the word 'fat', and the only way to really describe them would require the invention of a new word. I collected all the information the truth beam had gathered over time. Then I looked at information collected by weight loss programs to see what words fat people used to describe themselves.

Wow! This was very encouraging!

The truth beam showed me that almost every fat person had tried to lose weight at least once - most fat people didn't really like being fat!  And, the reasons they wanted to lose weight had now supplied the foundation for the new word:

Sad      (Yes, being fat made them unhappy.)

Pathetic (Fat people said that letting themselves get in that state really was pathetic.)

Ugly/Disgusted   (Fat people said they felt ugly.  When they took a good look in the mirror they were disgusted with their bodies.)

This was perfect!  I had created a word that was actually inspired by fat people themselves!  'SPUD!'

"Oh, no, Lamp!  By granting that third wish I started something that is completely out of control.  I am responsible for this!  Everyone is getting fatter and fatter and becoming SPUDs."

Something had to be done, but I didn't know what!  Once a wish has been granted it can't be taken back or changed. I had gotten carried away with that lie and given an endless, fast, convenient supply of fatty food to a couple of sprogs, and now *everyone* was eating it!  I asked Lamp if he had any ideas.

"You need to explain to everyone that eating too much will make them fat and that they shouldn't eat it," said Lamp.

I reminded Lamp about the conversation with the kids. "Don't you remember, Lamp? Humans lie to themselves all the time. Telling the truth causes them upset and pain so they just pretend all the time."

"How is that possible?" said Lamp. "Surely they must see what they are doing to themselves. Look again at this picture."

The picture showed men with big, ugly-looking, saggy bellies hanging over their swim shorts, and women wearing stuff that made you want to rip your eyes out! I saw fat squeezing out of all sorts of places. It was horrible. "But look, Lamp, they are all smiling, eating, drinking and laughing, and not a bit worried about the way they look or how unhealthy they are."

How strange, I thought. "Maybe we do have it all wrong, Lamp." Lamp had an idea. He asked me to send a truth beam into one of the fat people to find out what they were really feeling.

I went to the beach and looked for very fat people. I didn't have to look far. I saw one bloke standing in the water. His belly was huge and his chest was saggy. He looked perfectly happy, though, so I thought I would look around for someone else.

"No, Genie," said Lamp, "fire your truth beam at *him*."

"Ok, here goes." My beam hit the fat bloke and bounced right back with the results.    "The beam must not be working, Lamp.    It shows nothing at all."

"Fire it deeper, Genie.  Remember, you are only seeing what is on the surface," said Lamp.

This time the beam went right under his skin.    It took a little longer to come back. "Oh dear, Lamp, you are right!  It says that he is embarrassed about being fat but puts on an act to hide it.    He believes that there is nothing he can do about it, so he just calls himself a big guy and now lies his way through each day."

Lamp said, "Genie, fire the beam at him one more time, only this time go deeper, right into his soul, a place where nothing can hide, a place where real emotions are felt. Then we will know for sure what is *really* going on."

One last time, I fired the beam as deep as it could go, and waited. A few minutes passed; the beam started to return. Only this time it was very slow and very heavy, struggling to get back to me. After a few more minutes, the beam was back and there it was! Just as we had thought all along! The truth beam had gone deep into his soul and found anger, misery and incredible embarrassment. It uncovered great sadness and low self-esteem. This was a man who was living a self-imposed prison sentence, shackled to a lie from which it was impossible to break free. His huge gut had become what defined him; he had become accustomed to being called the 'Big Man'. His fatness was now his complete identity.

"Genie, is there anything we can do to help this chap get back on track?" Lamp was concerned, worried about this guy and desperate to help him. I told Lamp that the truth beam indicated he was actually beyond help. His lifestyle was now set in stone.
The changes he needed to make were far too vast and complicated because the truth was buried so deep in his soul. He would never, ever see it. Even the truth beam had struggled to get there.

"We can only help those people who have the truth lying close to the surface and unfortunately, most fat adults are in the same boat as this chap."

Lamp had another idea. "Genie, you need to find the kids you gave all that food to when you granted that third wish. They are, of course, adults now, but that was when everyone started to overeat.  Hopefully, we can find people who are not too fat and can be helped."

I used my genie magic and located the kids who, as Lamp said, were now adults, and as feared, many were indeed very fat. I wasted no time firing the truth beam, and waited for the results to come back.  But, just like the chap on the beach, almost all of those kids had eaten their way into misery. Penetrating once again deep into their souls, the truth beam unearthed what had to be the most devastating truth of all: fat adults are doomed.  It's too late… there was no fixing this.

"How can this be true?" asked Lamp. "Surely we can do something?"

"No, Lamp, there is nothing anyone can do. A person has a free will to make their own choices, and only that person can choose to do what is necessary. Fat people live a fat person's life and getting them to change their entire life is an impossible task."

"Genie, you are wrong. I have seen TV commercials that promise weight loss, fat loss, six-pack abs, and more. I've even seen an ad for a blanket with sleeves that looked very snugly and I'd like to get one!"

"No, Lamp, that is just humans lying again. Remember, humans lie to themselves and to others. The people on the commercials are professional liars and the people who buy from the commercials are so desperate they will believe anything." Lamp looked very upset and I saw a tear in his eye. "Don't let it get you down, Lamp. We can still save the children. Most of them are not fat yet."

"Oh, no, Genie, I'm upset because I wanted a Snuggie®!"

"Lamp, I'll get you one, but first things first! We need a plan to save the kids." It was then I realized we had found all the kids but one... Freddy. We hadn't found Freddy. "Lamp, we need to find Freddy. He has to be around here somewhere." We searched every house in the city until we came to a little cottage standing all alone. I peeked through the window and there he was... Freddy! It was that little, fat kid all grown up. But wait, he wasn't fat... well, yes, he *was* fat and out of shape, but nothing like all the other fat people. I wonder... I thought to myself. I fired the truth beam at Freddy, and the beam bounced right back. Fantastic! The truth was just below his skin! We can save Freddy! He is unhappy with his weight but aware that he is responsible for being fat. He has tried many times to lose weight and is close to believing that it is an impossible task. But, Freddy was not yet a SPUD!

"See, Lamp, this is what happens. There appears to be a sequence, starting with 'I'm fat, but I will lose it some day'. After getting fatter, that changes to, 'There must be something wrong with me, I just can't lose weight'.

This is when they become prey for the infomercial liars. After the 'money-back guarantee' promises fail, they look in the mirror and accept that this is 'just the way I'm meant to be'. Once someone reaches fat acceptance, they are lost forever. They become SPUDs. Freddy is not at the acceptance stage yet. "Look, Lamp, there is one of those abdominal pulsating, get-a-six-pack-without-exercise belt things, that do absolutely nothing except sting and burn your skin. Can you see it, Lamp? It is sitting on that stack of workout DVD's.  Obviously, Freddy has been trying. Lamp, are you listening to me?" I looked at Lamp.  He was staring into Freddy's window, mouth open wide, eyes transfixed as though hypnotized.

"Lamp, what is it?"

"I see a Snuggie®!"

"Lamp, I said I would get you one!"

I knew what had to be done.  I had to get Freddy to look a bit deeper, to get him to see that every day he is closer to becoming a SPUD.  He needed to completely change direction.

"Lamp, I have got it! I am going to wait until Freddy falls asleep and I'm going in. I am going to control his dream.

I waited, watching Freddy eat his dinner. It was like watching someone who was maxed out on their credit card handing over that card to purchase a big screen TV. Freddy was in FAT debt; he was maxed out. Adding to that debt made him feel good in the moment, but actually he, like the big screen TV buyer, was really buying misery. Showing Freddy how unhealthy being fat is would not work. He hears that message everyday, in the same way that smokers hear it, too. That doesn't make them quit.

As I waited for Freddy to fall asleep, I thought about smokers...Why would a beautiful woman spend hours doing her hair, applying make-up, and perfume, trying on outfit after outfit until she feels she looks just right… and then, totally destroy the whole process by making herself smell exactly the same as an ashtray?!   Really, what's that all about? Maybe someone should just tell her the truth:  she stinks!   Maybe then she would quit!

**That was it!**

Instead of focusing on the health problems of being fat maybe people need to hear 'The Truth'. Lamp pointed out a problem with that idea. "Genie I only need one example," said Lamp. "Honey, does my bum look fat in these jeans"?

I know I can be a bit dumb at times, but I didn't know what Lamp was talking about.   Lamp explained that a woman often asks her man how she looks, and the man will always say she looks great. "Even if she looks like she has a month's worth of groceries stuffed in her pants?" I asked. Lamp nodded.

It was obvious to me that "The Truth" was *really* the only way to go, as everything else had failed. There are thousands of diet books on the shelves, and even more workout DVD's and internet fitness sites that are available twenty-four hours a day, seven days a week, but everyone is still getting fatter.

"No Lamp, I think the only way is to use 'The Truth'".

I fired the truth beam at Freddy one more time, this time looking to see if he cared what other people thought. The beam came back immediately with a very strong message: **all humans care**

**what others think, but they work hard to pretend they don't**.

This was very exciting because I now knew the remedy. I had figured out a way to solve the problem of obesity! Lamp was right though, a man telling his lady that her bum looks like it's getting ready to explode would not make him very popular. This was a massive roadblock. If 'The Truth' was going to be the weapon of choice, we needed a way to deliver it. But, it was very clear that humans are incapable of hitting a loved one with such a devastating blow. I on the other hand, don't have any trouble telling someone that they are FAT.

So the stage was set and it was time for action; this was a serious problem that needed a no nonsense approach. From now on I am the Fit Genie who tells people to **STOP BEING FAT!**

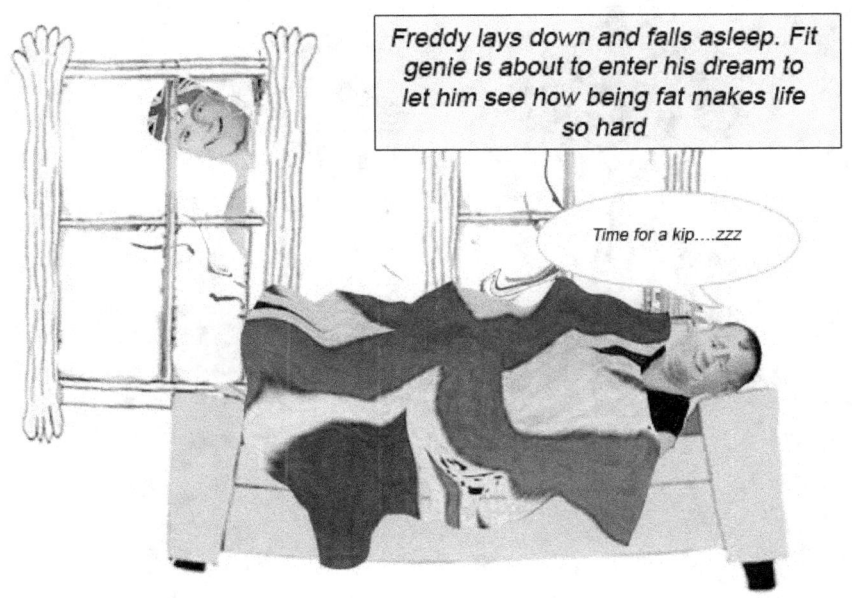

Freddy was now sleeping.   Time to put my plan into action!

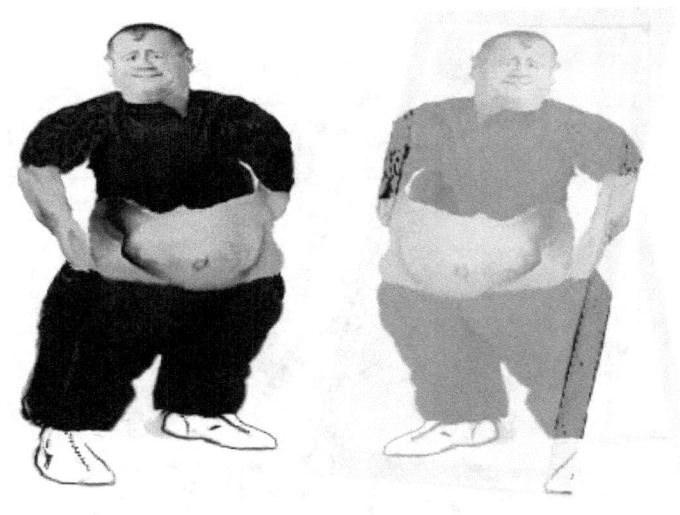

I went into Freddy's dream and took control; in his dream Freddy thought he had woken up. He stood up and made his way to his bedroom. He looked in the mirror and could see his belly hanging over his pants. I had made his belly *a little bit* bigger.

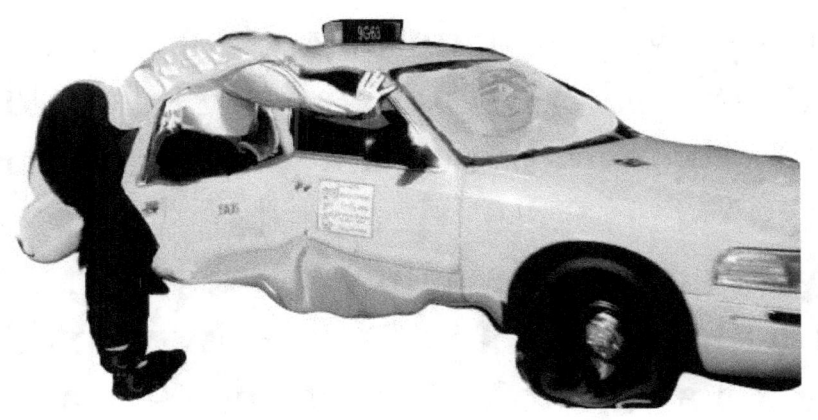

Freddy then found himself in a taxicab on the way to the airport. The taxi driver asked Freddy if he was going to a fatty's convention. Freddy noticed he was now even fatter than before, and that people were staring at him.

Freddy found himself in line to board a plane. He was very self-conscious, as people pointed, laughed and made jokes about him. A baggage handler told him he would have to go in the hold with the cargo, as he would not fit in a plane seat.

Freddy was now in the plane sitting with the other passengers. He could hear them talking about him, and making fat jokes. He heard one person say, 'can you imagine what he must look like in his undies?' Freddy wanted to hide away, so he closed his eyes and pretended this wasn't happening. When he opened his eyes, he was on a beautiful beach surrounded by beautiful people; couples playing volleyball, others jet-skiing and parasailing. Now Freddy was even fatter.

His clothes hardly covered him. He felt embarrassed beyond belief and just wanted to get away and hide. He looked around. There were no other fat people in sight. He stood out like a sore thumb. He looked down and saw the lamp. He knew he had seen this lamp before somewhere, so he picked it up. As he held the lamp, I spoke to him.

"Freddy, we need to have a chat," I said. I came out of the lamp and asked Freddy to cast his mind back to the time when he and his friends were given three wishes. They were warned what would happen if they ate too much. Freddy was dying inside. Having so many people laughing at him was just too much for him to take. I asked Freddy if he remembered what I had offered for his last wish, but he had chosen to turn down. He said he did remember and that he thought about that every day of his life. Finding out that people were making fun of him behind his back was what made him try to lose the weight to begin with. I then told Freddy the offer still stands, that I could make him fit, slim and healthy but he would not stay that way unless he ate right and exercised regularly.

Freddy started to cry, "Yes, oh yes, please, I will do anything, just get me out of this fat, disgusting body. I can't do fat anymore!" So, with a blink of an eye, Freddy was slim, fit, muscular and very healthy.

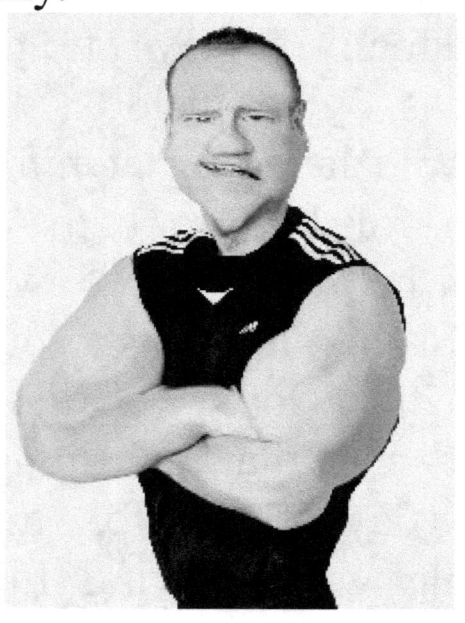

He ran down the beach and joined in all the fun. I asked Freddy if he would join me to help other fat people lose their weight and get into shape. He said he would be delighted. I told him it was not going to be easy, so he best get a little rest.

Freddy lay down in the warm sand and fell asleep. When he awoke, his dream was over and he was back home. He got up and looked in the mirror. He saw that it had all been just a dream and he was back in his fat body. He saw something glimmering in the corner. It was the lamp. He picked it up and I spoke to him. This time it was not a dream.

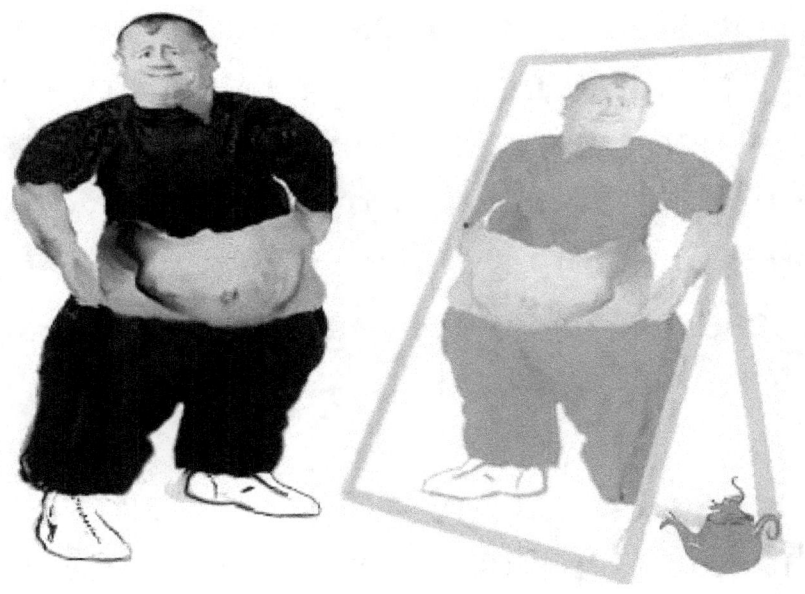

"Freddy," I said, "I have discovered the cure for obesity. It's not for sale on an infomercial, and you won't find it in any magic pill.  The cure is free, and available to everyone immediately. But, it starts with accepting 'The Truth'.  If 'The Truth' was actually a pill it would be the bitterest pill you would ever have to swallow."

"Freddy, 'The Truth' is you are fat and out of shape, people make jokes about you and call you fatty behind your back. Your clothes are those you have to put up with and not what you want to wear. You look disgusting and the thought of touching your fat is quite repulsive and puke-inducing to most people.   Just because you've been ignoring it, doesn't mean it is not true."

"These are not my words.  These are the thoughts I collected from the truth beam when fired into the majority of the human population.   These thoughts even came from other fat people: they see people fatter than themselves as disgusting, too. The cure only works for those people who care what other people think. For those who truly don't, there is no cure, as they don't even care about themselves.

Freddy was ready. He wanted the fit, healthy body that I had given him a taste of in his dream. I couldn't just hand it to him in reality though. He had to work for it, like everyone else.

'The Truth' was going to be our most powerful tool in battling obesity. The biggest battle would be getting humans to accept it!

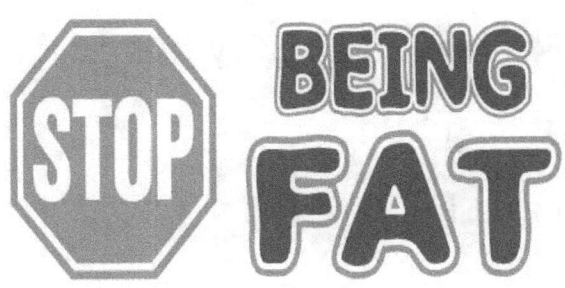

*Yes! It's a choice!*

# *Fit Genie Lingo Dictionary*

- bloke - man
- bum – bottom; derriere
- butcher's – to look at, as in "take a butcher's"
- chap - guy
- chin wag – a discussion
- deaf and dumb – bum
- git – a silly, stupid person
- heff – a very fat person
- kip – a nap
- lumbered – burdened with; stuck with
- plonker – really, really dumb
- sprog – a child
- Tom and Dick – sick
- wicked – awesome

www.ingramcontent.com/pod-product-compliance
Lightning Source LLC
Chambersburg PA
CBHW060225290526
45789CB00003B/1410